PRE TEEN PRESSURES

AIDS

by Paula McGuire

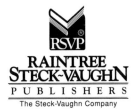

RSVP

RAINTREE
STECK-VAUGHN
PUBLISHERS
The Steck-Vaughn Company

Austin, Texas

Consultants
Scott Moyer, Consortium Coordinator, Mercer County HIV Consortium, Trenton, NJ
William B. Presnell, Clinical Member, American Association for Marriage and Family Therapy

Developed for Steck-Vaughn Company by
Visual Education Corporation, Princeton, New Jersey
Project Director: Jewel Moulthrop
Editorial Assistant: Jacqueline Morais
Photo Research: Sara Matthews
Electronic Preparation: Cynthia C. Feldner, Manager; Elaine Weiss
Production Supervisor: Ellen Foos
Electronic Production: Lisa Evans-Skopas, Manager; Elise Dodeles, Deirdre Sheean, Isabelle Verret
Interior Design: Maxson Crandall

Raintree Steck-Vaughn Publishers staff
Editor: Kathy DeVico
Project Manager: Joyce Spicer

Photo Credits: Cover: © Tom McCarthy/PhotoEdit; 6: © Tony Freeman/PhotoEdit; 8: © Richard Cash/PhotoEdit; 12: © Jeff Greenberg/PhotoEdit; 13: © David Young-Wolff/PhotoEdit; 16: © Tom McCarthy/PhotoEdit; 18: © David Boe/UPI/Corbis-Bettmann; 20: © Guy Gillette/Photo Researchers, Inc.; 24: © Myrleen Ferguson Cate/PhotoEdit; 26: © Michael Newman/PhotoEdit; 28: © David Young-Wolff/PhotoEdit; 31: © Jonathan Nourok/PhotoEdit; 32: © Bob Padgett/Reuters/Corbis-Bettmann; 35: © David Young-Wolff/PhotoEdit

Library of Congress Cataloging-in-Publication Data
McGuire, Paula.
    AIDS/by Paula McGuire.
        p.   cm. — (Preteen pressures)
    Includes bibliographical references and index.
    Summary: Explains what HIV and AIDS are, how the virus is spread, the importance of testing, and how to cope with the disease.
    ISBN 0-8172-5025-5
    1. AIDS (Disease)—Juvenile literature. 2. AIDS (Disease) in children—Juvenile literature. [1. AIDS (Disease) 2. Diseases.]   I. Title. II. Series.
RC607.A26M388 1998
616.97′92—dc21   97-22366
                                                         CIP
                                                         AC

Printed and bound in the United States
  2 3 4 5 6 7 8 9 0 LB 01 00 99

CONTENTS

INTRODUCTION

Nearly everybody knows that AIDS has become a worldwide epidemic—a rapidly spreading disease that is difficult to control. You probably have heard about famous people in sports and entertainment who have AIDS. You may have seen programs on TV to raise money for AIDS research. You certainly hear about AIDS from the news, and most kids learn something about it in school.

AIDS first became known in the United States in 1981, so American doctors and researchers—people who look for the answers to medical problems—have not had a very long time to study it. They may never know where or how it began. Some people believe that the disease had been in the United States, Europe, and Africa for a long time.

So far, no cure for AIDS has been found. We know that AIDS comes from a virus—a microscopic organism that causes disease. The AIDS virus is called HIV (Human Immunodeficiency Virus). Almost everybody who is infected with HIV eventually develops AIDS and dies.

Here are some facts about AIDS in the world:

▶ The World Health Organization (WHO) estimates that as of mid-1995, 18.5 million people, including 1.5 million children, were infected with HIV, the virus that causes AIDS.

▶ WHO states that a total of 1,169,811 AIDS cases were reported as of June 30, 1995, a 19 percent increase over those reported up to July 1, 1994.

- In 1993 AIDS killed more young people than did any other infectious disease.
- AIDS is the third leading cause of death in the United States among men and women between the ages of 25 and 44.

For the moment, as you can see, most of the news about AIDS is bad. However, some progress has been made. Medicines have been discovered that can help people who have AIDS and prolong their lives. Also, the sooner you start learning about the disease, the better off you are. AIDS is passed from person to person, mostly through certain kinds of risky behavior. Preteens and teens can have the disease, just as adults can. Because of AIDS, people of all ages throughout the world have changed—or should change—the ways they think and act. There is no longer a choice if you want to avoid having AIDS.

Reading this book is a good way to begin to understand the disease. The facts you need are here. If you have questions or fears about what you read, share them with your friends, parents, teachers, or doctors. The more you talk about AIDS with others, the more you'll learn. And the more you know, the better you can protect yourself. Until doctors can find a way to cure the disease, knowing the facts about AIDS is the best way to keep yourself healthy.

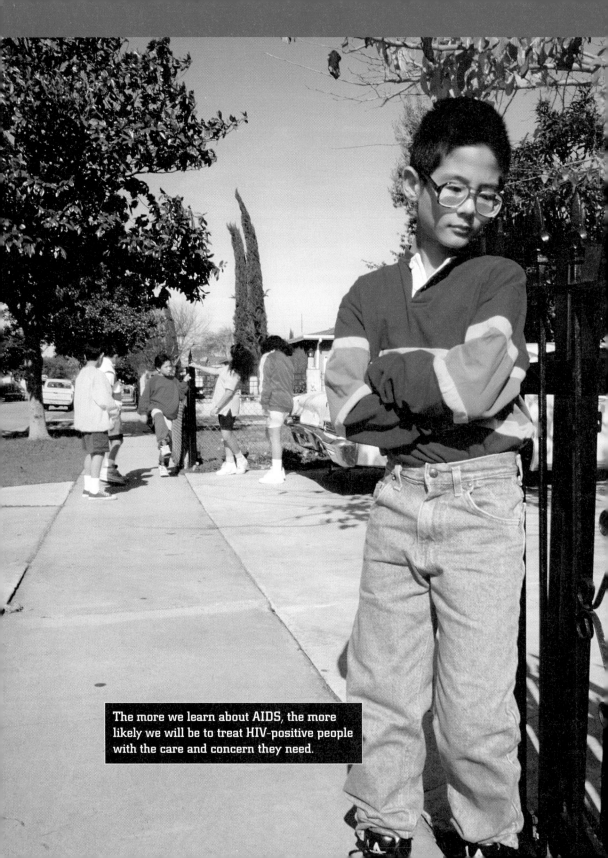

The more we learn about AIDS, the more likely we will be to treat HIV-positive people with the care and concern they need.

HIV AND AIDS

66My name is Pete. A new kid moved to our street a few weeks ago. I saw him the day his family moved in. He looked sort of pale and skinny, and I didn't see him again for a while.

We play baseball in the lot across the street, and he finally came out one day and hung around the backstop. We said hello, and he smiled. He said his name was Danny, but he didn't feel like playing. He seemed a little sad.

Later, when I went home, my mom said that I shouldn't play with Danny. I asked her why, and she said that she heard Danny has AIDS.

'How could he have AIDS?' I asked. 'He's only a kid.'

'Well, I'm not sure how he got it, but you stay away from him. You might catch it, too.'**99**

Actually, Pete's mother is wrong. Danny doesn't have AIDS. He is HIV-positive. That means that the virus that causes AIDS has entered his bloodstream. He has become infected, but he is not yet sick with the disease.

Pete also has a mistaken idea about AIDS. He thinks that kids can't have AIDS. Nearly 7,000 children in the United States have AIDS.

Many people don't know the facts about HIV and AIDS. It is true that a person who is infected with HIV almost always develops the disease called AIDS. Medical researchers are working hard to find a cure for

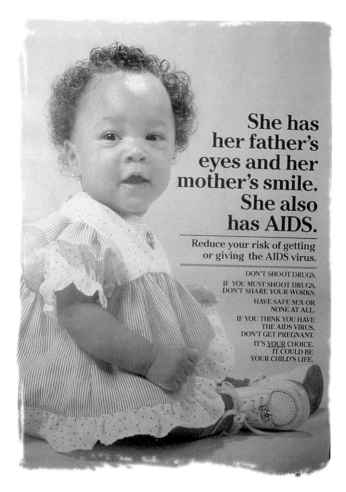

Posters are one way of educating people about HIV and AIDS. They usually include a telephone number to call for more information.

AIDS, but as yet there is none. There are several ways to become infected, so it is important for people to know all they can about HIV and AIDS. Then they will not be so scared. They will also better understand the people who do have AIDS, and maybe save some hurt feelings.

HIV

You have probably heard the word *virus* before. A virus is a microscopic organism that enters the bloodstream and causes diseases. Flu viruses cause the flu. You often hear people who are sick with the flu say that they "have a virus." HIV is the name of the virus that causes AIDS. HIV is a shorter way of saying the medical term *Human Immunodeficiency Virus.*

People's blood can be tested for HIV. If the virus is present, the person is said to be HIV-positive. When a person becomes HIV-positive, it means that the virus is attacking the body's immune system. The immune system is the body's defense against disease. It fights germs that can enter the body and helps you stay healthy. It also helps you recover when you are sick.

The body's immune system has special white blood cells. They are called T cells, and they help protect the body from illness. When HIV attacks the body, the T cells fight the virus for a while. But HIV is very strong, and it finally weakens and destroys the T cells. The body is then, in medical terms, immunodeficient. That's another way of saying that the body is without a defense system, or that it has no way to fight disease.

AIDS

When the body becomes defenseless, a disease may easily attack and take over. A person with too few T cells can become sick with one or more diseases called AIDS-related diseases. Two of these diseases, pneumonia and tuberculosis, affect the lungs. Another disease affects the skin. There are about 26 AIDS-related diseases. When an HIV-positive person has one of these diseases or has a low number of T cells, he or she is considered to have AIDS.

In other words, AIDS develops when a person who is HIV-positive can no longer resist disease. Furthermore, a person who is HIV-positive almost always comes down with an AIDS-related disease sooner or later. It may take many years, but Danny will almost certainly develop AIDS one day.

AIDS is a shorter way of saying a longer medical term. Here is a way to help you remember what the letters mean:

ACQUIRED
Something that was picked up.

IMMUNO
Referring to the body's immune system.

DEFICIENCY
A lack, or not enough, of something.

SYNDROME
A group of symptoms, or warning signs, in the body.

The AIDS Story in Numbers

The total number of AIDS cases reported in the United States (1981–1994) was 427,392.

Reported by age:	
Under 5 years old:	4,711
5 to 12 years old:	1,184
13 to 29 years old:	78,838
30 to 39 years old:	195,304
40 to 49 years old:	103,894
50 to 59 years old:	31,319
Over 60 years old:	12,142

Sources: U.S. Centers for Disease Control and Prevention, Atlanta, GA; *Health United States 1993,* National Center for Health Statistics, U.S. Dept. of Health and Human Services.

Total deaths in the United States from AIDS (1982–1994) were 258,658, including 850 persons who were 13 to 19 years old and 44,770 who were 20 to 29 years old.

Since it is estimated that on the average it takes 10 years before a person who is HIV-positive develops an AIDS-related disease, most of the persons in the second group (ages 20 to 29) were infected during their teenage years.

AVOIDING THE CONFUSION

You may be happy to learn that it is not as easy to catch HIV as it is to catch a cold. You can become infected with a cold virus by sitting next to someone in class who is coughing and sneezing. Unlike other viruses, HIV cannot live in the air. It cannot infect air, food, or water.

HOW HIV IS NOT SPREAD

HIV is <u>not</u> spread by casual contact. A person cannot catch HIV from:

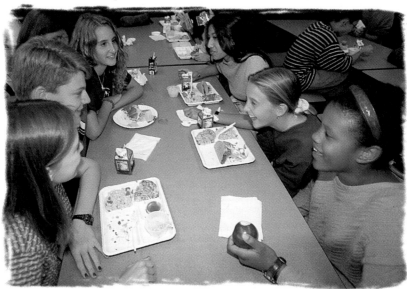

AIDS cannot be spread through sharing food.

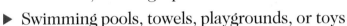

AIDS cannot be spread through drinking fountains.

▶ Going to school or working with an infected person; or using an infected person's pencil, book, or telephone

▶ Mingling in a crowd, eating in a restaurant or a school cafeteria, drinking from a water fountain, touching a doorknob, or using a public toilet

▶ Swimming pools, towels, playgrounds, or toys

▶ Shaking hands or touching someone

▶ Friendly kissing

▶ Giving blood in hospitals for sick people

▶ Mosquito bites

HOW HIV IS SPREAD

Any discussion of HIV or AIDS has to include sex and drugs. These subjects may make you feel uncomfortable or embarrassed. Some parents, too, may not like to discuss sex or drugs, whether for moral, religious, or personal reasons. However, parents always want to protect their children. And more and more parents now agree that <u>not</u> talking about AIDS may be dangerous for their children. Sex and drugs are the two main causes of HIV infection in preteens and teens. Therefore, it is very important to know the basic facts.

The Office of National AIDS Policy estimates that:

► One of every four new HIV infections in the United States happens among young people under the age of 20

► Between 40,000 and 80,000 Americans become infected with HIV each year, an average of 110 to 220 a day

► Between 27 and 54 American young people become infected each day, or more than 2 young people every hour

► More than 7 million people in the world between the ages of 15 and 24 have been infected with HIV; many of them have already died

HIV is passed from person to person. The AIDS virus cannot live outside the body, and human skin is a good barrier against it. HIV lives in blood, semen (the male fluid that carries sperm), and vaginal secretions. To pass from one person to another, HIV must be carried by one of these body fluids from inside one person to inside another.

SEMEN AND VAGINAL FLUIDS

HIV is in the blood, semen (whether leaked or ejaculated), or vaginal fluids of an infected person. If an infected person has sexual intercourse, HIV can enter the other person's body through the vagina, penis, rectum, or mouth. If sores or cuts are present, especially during anal sex (through the rectum) or oral sex (by mouth), the sexual act is particularly risky.

Sexual intercourse may be made safer by the use of a latex condom. A condom is a covering for the penis that traps the semen and prevents it from entering another person's body. You may have heard the term *safer sex*. This refers to using a condom and preventing fluids from entering someone else's body. Using a condom reduces the risk of spreading infection. It also helps avoid an unwanted pregnancy. Not using a condom is "unprotected" sex and is very risky behavior.

BLOOD

Sometimes a person needs to receive blood from another person. This is called a blood transfusion. Blood transfusions are needed when a person has been in an accident, has a serious illness, or needs surgery.

People who have hemophilia need frequent transfusions. Hemophilia is a disorder in which a person's blood does not clot, or thicken, properly. People who have this disorder can bleed uncontrollably, even from the smallest cut. They can be helped through transfusions of blood that contains a special clotting factor called antihemophilic factor (AHF). AHF is gathered from many units of blood plasma (the clear, liquid part of blood).

Many people donate, or give, their blood to blood banks or to hospitals where blood is stored for use when necessary. There is no risk of becoming infected with HIV from donating blood. The needles that hospitals and blood banks use to draw blood come in sterile packages and are never used again.

Although donating blood is safe, receiving blood from a person who has HIV is very dangerous. HIV can be passed on by a transfusion of an infected person's blood into someone else's body. People who think that they may have behaved in a risky way even once should not donate blood.

All blood that is donated in the United States is now tested for HIV. Unfortunately, before the virus was discovered, many people received infected blood from transfusions. Thousands of people with hemophilia became infected with HIV. And there is still a small risk, since people may donate blood before signs of infection show up on a test.

Sometimes it can take as long as six months for the infection to show up in a blood test. Now many people who are going to have surgery donate their own blood beforehand. Then, if they need a transfusion during surgery, their own blood is available.

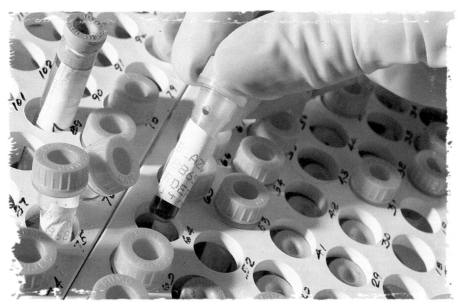

All donated blood in the United States is now tested for HIV before it is used.

DRUGS

Injecting drug use (IDU) directly involves blood. What happens is that some blood is drawn back into the needle when it is pulled out of the skin. If that needle is used again, the blood in the needle passes into the bloodstream of the next person. If the first person was HIV-positive, the next person can become infected, too.

Recent studies show an increase in the use of non-injectable drugs (including marijuana, cocaine, and alcohol) among young people. The use of these drugs impairs judgment and can lead to risky drug-related and sexual behavior. This is especially true of young people, who are naturally curious, like to experiment, and think that no harm can come to them. Any drug use, however, can put their lives and welfare at risk.

HAVING BABIES

Around 25 percent of pregnant women who are infected with HIV pass on the infection to their babies. A baby may become infected in the uterus before birth or during birth.

All babies from HIV-infected mothers test positive for the virus at birth. This is because a baby is born with its mother's immune system. At about 18 months of age, when a baby develops its own immune system, the baby may test negative. The baby also can become infected with HIV from breast-feeding. For this reason, many doctors in the United States recommend that an infected mother give her baby formula instead of breast milk.

The Case of Ryan White

In 1990 Ryan White, a young man from Kokomo, Indiana, died of AIDS. He was 18 years old. Ryan was diagnosed HIV-positive when he was 13, just about the same age as Danny, the boy discussed by Pete and his mom earlier in this book. Danny

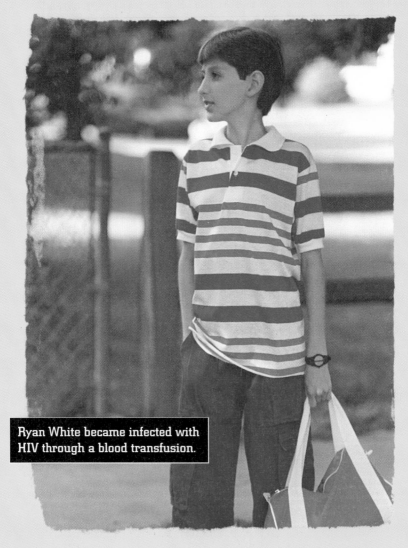

Ryan White became infected with HIV through a blood transfusion.

does not have hemophilia as Ryan did, but both boys were infected by contaminated blood during a transfusion.

At the time Ryan was infected, AIDS had just been discovered. No one was sure how it was transmitted. Because people were so fearful and confused about the disease, they were cruel and unkind to Ryan and his family.

Back in the mid-1980s, people didn't want HIV-positive students in public school. The local school system tried to keep Ryan out. Ryan and his mother fought a long legal battle for his right to be in school. The townspeople were unfriendly and often insulted them.

At last Ryan was allowed to attend school under certain conditions. He had to use separate eating utensils and a separate bathroom. He could not drink from the water fountains in the hallway. He was not allowed in the gym or in the swimming pool. The building was disinfected every night.

Almost half the students stayed away from school to protest Ryan's presence. People picketed the school, and someone fired a gunshot through the Whites' living room window. Finally the Whites moved to another town.

Because of his brave struggle, Ryan became a nationally known figure and won the sympathy of many people. Olympic diving champion Greg Louganis gave his winning medal to Ryan. Pop star Elton John flew Ryan to Disneyland. Ryan also was a guest on the "Tonight" show on TV. He made many public appearances—including one before the Presidential Commission on AIDS—to speak about AIDS before he died. Ryan White is remembered by everybody as a courageous fighter.

Today much more is known about AIDS, and many people have become more reasonable in their response to the disease. Danny—and other young people like him—may not have to suffer during their last years as much as Ryan White did.

Each year about 7,000 babies are born to HIV-positive mothers. Of those children, 54 percent will be diagnosed with AIDS by the time they are seven years old. Most will become orphans when their mothers, and often their fathers, die from the disease.

TEENS ARE AT RISK

According to the Centers for Disease Control (CDC), 1 in 5 AIDS cases in the United States is diagnosed in people between 20 and 29 years of age. It is important to understand that on the average it takes ten years for AIDS to develop in an HIV-positive person. Therefore, a majority of these AIDS cases resulted from HIV infections transmitted ten years earlier, when most of the persons were teenagers.

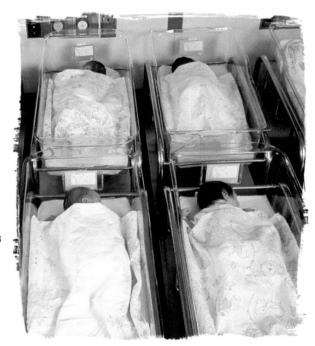

Over half of the babies born to HIV-positive mothers will be diagnosed with AIDS by the time they are seven years old.

YOU NEED TO KNOW THE FACTS

“My name is Shawna. I have an older brother, Jay, who lets me borrow pencils and stuff from his desk. One day when I opened the drawer, I found some condoms sort of hidden under some papers. I knew what they were right away. We had learned about them in Family Life class at school. It scared me that my brother had some, and I ran to get my mother.

Mom looked and just said, 'Oh.'

I didn't mean to be snooping. They were just there. 'Mom,' I said, 'what is he doing with those things?'

'Well, I have to say, this is kind of a surprise for me, too. Looks like he's thinking about having sex,' she said.

'But why is he doing that? Aren't you mad at him?'

Mom reminded me that Jay is 17, a lot older than I am. And that he's learned a lot of things that I'm just beginning to find out about.

'No,' she said. 'I guess I can't be mad at him. We've always tried to teach you kids the facts of life, and we've always trusted you to be responsible. Looks to me like he's doing just that.'

'But he's still just in high school!' I said.

Mom told me that maybe he'd never even used one. Maybe he was just keeping them around. Just in case. She told me she didn't think I should worry about this.

'Besides,' she said, 'this is Jay's business. I'm glad you came and told me what you found, but I think we should keep this conversation to ourselves. I'll always be around if you want to ask questions about anything. But I think Jay deserves his privacy. Just like you do. What do you say?'

I said she was right. Jay would die if he knew what I'd seen! 〞

Shawna's mother was able to give her daughter good advice at a difficult time. She understood that a pre-teen might be scared by suddenly finding evidence of a brother's sexual activity. On the other hand, she also had to admit that her teenage son was at least thinking about sex. And she respected his right to privacy. She invited Shawna to talk to her anytime. And she made Shawna feel better about what had just happened. It is important for preteens to have a parent, a friend, or an adviser who will answer questions openly and honestly.

Adolescence is the time when kids begin to notice changes in their bodies. These changes are part of general sexual development. Body parts not only change and grow but take on a different purpose and meaning. Preteens also begin to experience new feelings and emotions. Since these changes can sometimes cause confusion or unnecessary fears, let's talk about some of them.

Both boys and girls see changes in their bodies during their preteen years. Each person, however, develops at his or her own rate. Some girls begin developing breasts and growing hair on parts of their bodies by the time they are nine or ten. Some boys, too, grow hair, and their penises become larger sooner or later than their friends'.

CHANGES IN FEELINGS

Physical changes cause new sensations in parts of the body, sexual feelings that usually bring pleasure. If you or someone else touches certain parts of your body, for example, you may suddenly have surprisingly agreeable feelings.

Your responses are controlled as much by your emotions and memories as they are by physical sensations. Just being able to feel something doesn't mean you will necessarily feel sexual. Feeling sexual will depend in large part on what's going on at the moment—the mood you're in, the person you're with, and where you are.

Some preteens may also feel eager for sexual contact with someone else. They want to experience the new feelings they are learning about. They are the ones who most enjoy playing kissing games and turning out the lights at parties. However, they may not understand that others do not feel the same way. This can cause problems for people who still feel like little kids inside of growing bodies. They may feel scared if they are rushed about their sexual feelings.

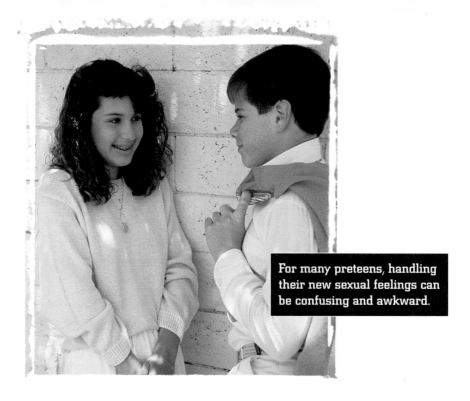

For many preteens, handling their new sexual feelings can be confusing and awkward.

Some preteens are happy just to think about sex. They imagine all sorts of wonderful things, perhaps kissing or touching someone, or not doing anything but just thinking about a special person. It is having the warm or close feeling with someone that many people think is important, not necessarily the sexual experience itself. So learning about these new feelings may be different for each person. Whatever your reactions to your own sexual feelings are, you can be sure that other kids around you are reacting to theirs, too.

Soon somebody will invite you to a boy-girl party or will ask you out on a date. You're going to have to figure out how you're going to behave. Knowing the difference between purely sexual feelings and your emotions is one of the most important lessons you can start to learn now.

DATING

It's not long before preteen boys and girls start looking at one another in a new and different way. As your bodies change, you just don't feel like chasing each other around or playing games the way you used to as little kids. Many preteens start dating by doing things in a group. Perhaps you'll find yourself attending a movie or a barbecue with a bunch of friends. This is a good way to meet people your age—to find out what other preteens talk about and how they act. Many of these friendships will continue through high school.

Sooner or later, however, you'll be all alone with somebody. It's often a scary situation for both people, but they generally get through it. You may become attracted to someone with whom you'll want to spend most of your time. Or you may prefer to date many different people. And it may well happen that you begin to feel sexually attracted to someone.

HOMOSEXUALITY

That "someone" could also be a person of the same sex. When you are attracted to someone of the same sex, it is called homosexuality. No one knows why a person is homosexual, or gay. Some people think that you are born that way. Others think that homosexuality is caused by the way you grew up. Still others think that you just want to be that way.

Homosexuality has been around for thousands of years. Sometimes it has been accepted by most people, sometimes not. Today many people are afraid of homosexuality. That is partly because, when AIDS was first recognized in the early 1980s, it seemed to occur mainly among homosexual men. However, now we know that sharing needles and having unprotected sex are the main causes of the spread of HIV, the virus that causes AIDS. Just being homosexual does not cause AIDS!

All this talk about homosexuality can be very confusing, especially if you are having trouble understanding

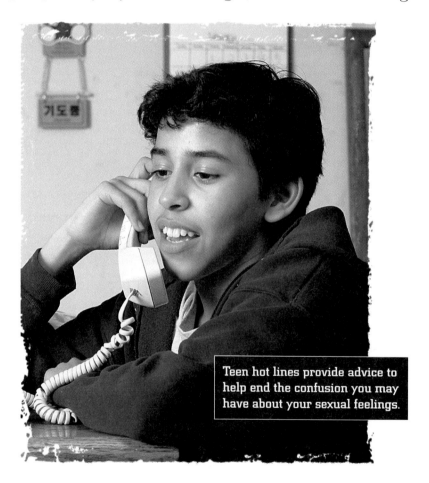

Teen hot lines provide advice to help end the confusion you may have about your sexual feelings.

your own feelings. If you think that you are gay, you may be feeling alone and afraid of being different from most people. It's important to find somebody to talk with about these feelings, but it may not be easy to find someone who is willing to discuss them with you. Nevertheless, you need to understand you're not alone in having such feelings. Many people feel just like you. Read books on the subject, talk to an adult or a friend if you can, or call a teen hot line. In time you will be able to think through your confusion and understand who you are.

READING THE ROAD SIGNS

We mentioned earlier that some preteens may feel eager for sexual contact. They especially may find it hard to resist the sexual messages of today's media. It is possible that a strong desire to have sex may make them lose control of their good sense. Imagine yourself, for example, jumping onto a bicycle without a helmet and racing down a steep hill without using your brakes! Letting your sexual feelings run away with you is very much the same thing. It is another example of very risky behavior. You've ignored the warning signs at the top of the hill: Danger! Steep Hill! Use Low Gear! You can have fun and excitement, but there is certainly danger ahead and possibly a bad accident. You should not take that chance if you know how to avoid it.

So, when holding hands and kissing turn into thinking about closer contact with your partner, it is time to be aware of the warning signs. It is especially important to avoid other kinds of risky behavior, such as drinking alcohol or using drugs. Sometimes the pressure to drink alcohol or take drugs is hard to resist. The trouble is that drinking and drug use can impair your judgment and make you do things that, deep down, you really don't want to—and know you should not do.

THINKING THINGS THROUGH

Thinking about "going all the way" is difficult enough without adding other risky behavior. Sexual intercourse is not something to race down the hill for. With

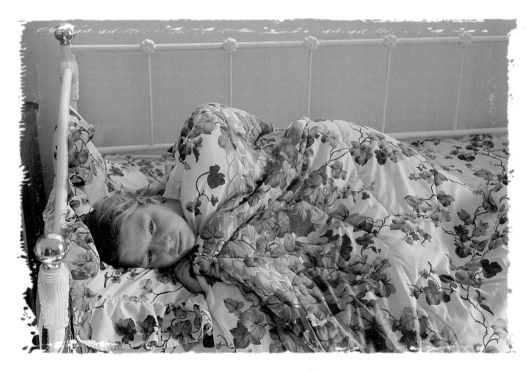

For those who drink alcohol or take drugs, the morning can be a painful time as they try to remember what happened the night before.

all the dangers ahead—becoming pregnant or becoming infected with HIV—it should be considered very carefully.

Those preteens who do have sex for the first time do so for many different reasons. Whatever the reason, these preteens have not paid attention to the warning signs. They may be heading for a crash.

PLAYING IT SAFE

Crashes come with regrets, shame, and disappointment. Too late, some preteens find that they were not ready for sex, or that it wasn't as pleasant as they thought it would be. Some feel that their partners took advantage of them. Some didn't practice "safer sex." They may be pregnant or infected with HIV or another sexually transmitted disease.

Crashes are never necessary. Take advantage now of the information that is available to you. Learn all you can about preventing pregnancy and disease. Avoid risky behavior, and ask for help from adults and older friends. Learn all you can about yourself, and make some decisions. It's OK to feel uncomfortable with the idea of having sex so young. It's OK to have religious or moral reasons against having sex at your age. It's OK to be afraid of becoming pregnant or infected with HIV. Whatever your reason, you are simply practicing abstinence—you are not "doing it" now. You are playing it safe and avoiding a crash that could ruin your life.

THE IMPORTANCE OF TESTING

If you believe that you are at risk of being HIV-positive because of something that happened, you should be tested for the virus. If the test is negative, you will have a chance to change your life. You can avoid the risks you've been taking. If the test is positive, you will have the chance to seek early treatment. Negative or positive, you have a chance to change your behavior and pay attention to your health.

If you've decided to be tested, tell your parents (or another adult whom you trust). They can help you find a doctor, a clinic, or a counseling center. People under 18 may need a parent's consent to be tested. But there are many organizations to go to for information about testing. Look in the back of this book for addresses and telephone numbers.

Two types of testing arrangements ensure your privacy. One type is confidential. That means that the test results are told only to you. The other type is anonymous. That means that you do not have to give your name. You are given a number, and the results are identified by that number only.

The test itself is called the ELISA test. If the ELISA test is positive, it is followed by a confirming Western Blot test. The tests search the blood for antibodies produced by the immune system to fight HIV. If a test finds these antibodies, you have tested positive. If not, you have tested negative. Even if you test negative now, if you have been involved in risky behavior recently, you should be tested again in six months. It takes the immune system up to six months to develop antibodies. It may be too soon now to find the antibodies in your blood.

It is most important for you to have counseling both before and after you are tested. You need to know what health care you can find if your test is positive. It is equally important for you to be educated about HIV, whatever the results of your test. You don't want to make the same mistake again. Don't think that you are immune forever from HIV. Take care of yourself. And if you think you need to be tested, don't let another day go by without telling someone.

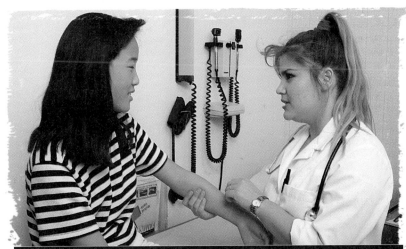

If you think you are HIV-positive, you should be tested. Many places offer HIV tests—doctors' offices, clinics, and counseling centers.

The Story of Magic Johnson

One person who wasn't concerned about risky behavior was Earvin "Magic" Johnson, the 32-year-old handsome, smiling, and inspiring point guard for the Los Angeles Lakers. Like other members of his team, Magic attracted the attention of female fans everywhere he traveled, and he was never at a loss for female companionship.

On the whole, the nation responded to Magic's announcement that he was HIV-positive with great support. People were learning that HIV could touch anyone. It was a human disease, after all, and those who were affected by it deserved understanding and respect.

Magic had no symptoms of AIDS. At first the doctors thought that continued play could harm his immune system, so Magic resigned from the team. This medical opinion changed, however, and he was soon back play-ing basketball for the Lakers. He also established the Magic Johnson Foundation to pro-mote medical care, education, and research on HIV and AIDS.

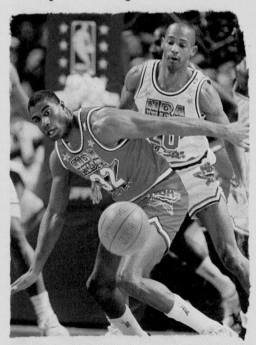

Magic went on to tell (with writer William Novak) his story to young readers in a book called *My Life*. Another book that he wrote is titled *What You Can Do to Avoid AIDS*. "If you don't know what you're doing about sex," he writes, "don't do it. Wait."

Magic Johnson went back to playing exhibition games with the Lakers. In 1992 he played in the NBA All-Star game and scored 25 points. He was named Most Valuable Player (MVP)—for the fourth time. "People with the virus can live on. Life doesn't stop because something happens to you," he said.

Some other players, however, objected to playing with Magic because he was HIV-positive. They were afraid that if he were injured during a game, they might become infected from contact with his blood. There was much argument about this, and Magic quit the Lakers again.

However, the 1992 International Olympics Committee ruled that HIV-positive athletes could compete in the 1992 games. Magic Johnson went to Barcelona, Spain, with the now-famous Gold Medal Dream Team. In 1994 he became a coach for the Lakers, and in February 1996 he began to play for them again.

At age 36, and 30 pounds heavier than he had been, Magic was still an outstanding player. In his first game, he scored 15 points. His health was good, and his attitude was positive. Still, a few months after rejoining the Lakers, he decided for the last time to quit playing basketball.

People wondered why he had quit. Most players and fans no longer worried very much about the possibility of being infected by an HIV-positive athlete. Medical opinion stated that the risk of infection was infinitesimal—very tiny. The CDC placed the risk at 1 in 85 million. And most people admired Magic's courage and his work for HIV and AIDS research.

Magic said that it was time for him to move on. Perhaps he was remembering what he had said a few years earlier: "I always wanted to be more than a basketball player, and I think I've become that. I've been dreaming of that all my life. And it took HIV to bring that out."

THE DISEASES OF AIDS

Some people may remain healthy for years after being infected with HIV. Others come down with a brief illness similar to the flu. Still others will not even know that they have the virus unless they are tested. The time when an infected person is not sick is called the asymptomatic period. Asymptomatic means without symptoms (signs) of illness.

The length of the asymptomatic period is different for each individual. It depends on whether the person eats and sleeps well, exercises regularly, and keeps his or her spirits high.

Staying well also depends on how much of the virus has entered the bloodstream and whether there is more than one kind of virus present. Even though a person may be asymptomatic, he or she can lose T cells.

THE APPEARANCE OF AIDS

AIDS occurs when an HIV-positive person becomes sick with an AIDS-related disease. The CDC says that an HIV-positive person has AIDS when he or she has a T-cell count of 200 or below. (The normal T-cell count is between 800 and 1,200.) Under normal conditions,

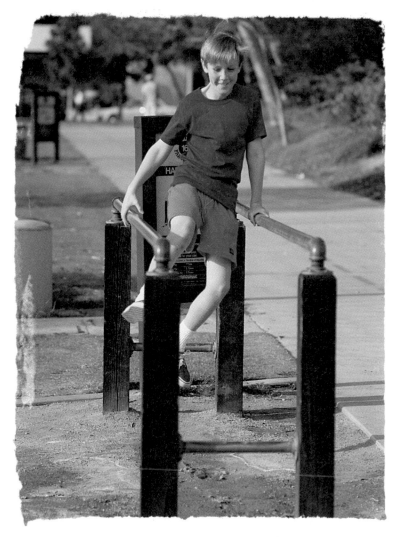

Regular exercise is an important part of remaining healthy after becoming infected with HIV.

an otherwise healthy person can fight an infection. Certain infections, however, seem to take the opportunity to make HIV-positive people sick. These opportunistic infections, or AIDS-related illnesses, seem to know that weakened immune systems can't fight back. One of these illnesses, alone or with others, will finally cause the death of a person who has lost too many T cells. We will describe a few of these illnesses.

A type of pneumonia known as PCP causes more deaths than any other AIDS-related illness. It is an infection of the lungs that usually causes a dry cough, fever, and shortness of breath. PCP can develop rapidly but can be treated if caught early enough.

Tuberculosis, or TB, is a common illness among people who have HIV. TB also affects the lungs. It is detected by a skin test, and most forms of the disease can be treated with medication.

Kaposi's sarcoma appears as purple or black sores that grow on the skin. Doctors once thought this disease was a type of cancer, but they now believe it is caused by another virus. The wounds can sometimes stop growing for a while, allowing people with the disease to live longer.

TREATMENT AND HOPE

For years doctors have been prescribing AZT (azidothymidine), a drug that has reduced the rate of deaths among people with AIDS. AZT can also delay the arrival of symptoms among those who are still healthy. It is usually prescribed when the T-cell count of a person infected with HIV falls below 500. The problem with AZT, however, is that within a year or two, the drug stops working. Until recently, there seemed to be no other way to control AIDS beyond this point.

Now, however, researchers know that AZT can help newborn babies whose mothers are HIV-positive—that is, if the mother was treated with AZT before giving birth. Tests have shown that the risk of transfer of HIV to the baby can be reduced by about two-thirds, from about 25 percent to about 8 percent. The mothers are also advised to avoid breast-feeding their infants.

Other gains have been made in slowing the progress of AIDS by using combinations of new and old drugs. Doctors are experimenting with several new drugs called protease inhibitors. These drugs show real promise in keeping HIV-positive people healthy and extending their lives. They do this by reducing the amount of HIV in patients' blood.

Although much remains to be done, these discoveries are encouraging. There is still no vaccine against HIV and no cure. Half of all HIV-positive people develop AIDS within 9 years of becoming infected, and 40 percent die within 10 years. And as long as people refuse to listen to the warnings about risky behavior, thousands may die before doctors can control the AIDS epidemic.

But there is another ray of hope. Doctors are discovering people who are HIV-positive but who have not developed AIDS. They have also found people who remain immune to infection despite repeated exposure to the virus. Some European babies born

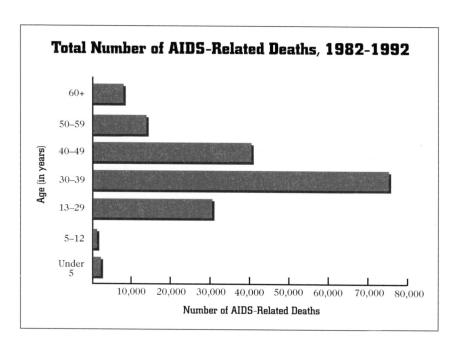

Total Number of AIDS-Related Deaths, 1982-1992

Age (in years)

- 60+
- 50–59
- 40–49
- 30–39
- 13–29
- 5–12
- Under 5

10,000 20,000 30,000 40,000 50,000 60,000 70,000 80,000

Number of AIDS-Related Deaths

Source: Statistical Abstract of the United States, 1996.

with HIV appear to be able to rid their systems of the virus. In Australia a small group of people received blood transfusions from an HIV-positive donor who was infected with the AIDS virus 15 years ago. So far, no one in the group has become ill. Neither has the person who donated the blood. Such cases are still rare. But researchers hope that by studying these people, they will find the key to better treatment and a cure.

COPING WITH AIDS

"I often wonder what my life would be like if I didn't have AIDS. I think my life may not have been much different.

But if I didn't have AIDS I would eat more and not be so skinny. I would not have to get needle sticks or take medicine that tastes sick. I would not have to get up at 11 P.M. or at 7 A.M. to take medicine and I would be able to eat whenever I wanted.

If I didn't have AIDS I would not have to worry about dying from it. My parents would probably be the same, though, whether or not I had AIDS. But if I didn't have AIDS they would not have to worry so much about me. It's hard for me to see my parents worry.

I often wonder how other children without AIDS learn to appreciate life. That's the best part about having AIDS."

—*Brett, Age 11*

People who have AIDS may take a long time to die. They need special care and attention from doctors and nurses and from their families. They may have to take many trips to a hospital and endure a long final stay. Since hospital care sometimes seems cold and un-friendly, some families prefer to keep a sick person at home. Others use the services of a hospice. A hospice may provide a team of doctors, nurses, home health aides, social workers, and chaplains. Hospice services are generally reserved for people who are not expected to live longer than six months.

FEELINGS ABOUT DEATH

When someone dies, especially a young person, people's emotions can take over their lives for a while. Some people feel anger—at doctors who couldn't save the sick person, at the lack of a cure for AIDS, at people who didn't show sympathy for AIDS patients, and at themselves for not being able to control their feelings. It's natural to feel anger and to question why this death occurred. But if you feel this way, you also need to learn how to turn your anger into positive actions. It is harm-ful to think about death too much or to let it take over your life.

Some people feel guilty about their past actions, or their behavior before the death occurred. It may have been hard for you to be near someone so sick. You may have complained about the person and now feel bad about having done that. Some people with AIDS still want to keep the disease a secret. Maybe you weren't told that the person was sick. You may have stayed away without meaning to ignore the situation. Now that the person has died, you may feel sorry that you didn't spend more time with him or her.

Above all, you may become sad and depressed after a death occurs. It is important to talk to people and let your feelings show. If you find that you are overwhelmed

> 66My mom has AIDS, and she's in the hospital most of the time. I don't like it when she's in the hospital. It scares me, because I never know if she's sick or not. I don't like it when she's sick. When she's sick I never know if she's going to die. I don't like to think of her dying because I don't want her to die. If she died the thing I would miss the most is her kisses and hugs. Right now, if I could tell my mom one thing it would be I LOVE YOU.
>
> P.S. I wish you didn't have AIDS and you could be with us forever. I will love you forever but if you're too tired to fight I'll still love you and it's OK. 99
>
> —*Mara, Age 9*

The essays by Brett and Mara were developed during therapeutic sessions with Lori S. Wiener of the National Cancer Institute, and excerpted from *Be a Friend: Children Who Live with HIV Speak* compiled by Lori S. Wiener, Ph.D., Aprille Best, and Philip A. Pizzo, M.D., © 1994 by Albert Whitman & Company. Reprinted by permission. All rights reserved.

by your feelings, tell a parent or another adult what is happening. This adult will help you find a way to understand your feelings and to live with your loss.

Always remember that anyone who has HIV or AIDS deserves your understanding and support.

WHAT YOU CAN DO IN THE FIGHT AGAINST AIDS

If you have been reading this book with care, you have learned a lot. You have learned important medical facts about the disease and about how many people have died of AIDS so far. You have learned about types of risky behavior and why it is important to avoid them.

For Yourself

Now that you are becoming sexually aware, you know that your actions and feelings need your careful attention. Don't do anything without thinking seriously beforehand. Make your decisions count. No one else owns your body; only you can keep your body safe and healthy. Don't abuse it or throw it away. Take good care of yourself. There's a wonderful world out there, and it's worth saving yourself for it.

For Others

Growing up sexually and learning about AIDS are already big jobs for a person. But when you think about it, they are not just jobs for you—they are for everybody. And there are ways that you can help others become aware of HIV and AIDS. Here is just a short list of activities to think about—taking part in just one can make a big difference to others:

▶ Continue to educate yourself and your friends about HIV and AIDS.

▶ Find out about the AIDS organizations in your community, and become a volunteer.

▶ Write or telephone national AIDS groups to find out how you can help with their activities.

▶ If you are curious about state or national policies on AIDS, write letters to your representatives in Congress.

Ask questions, state your opinions, and become involved. Ask your teachers for guidance, and suggest class projects. You can make a difference!

GLOSSARY

abstinence (sexual): Not having sexual intercourse.

AIDS: Acquired Immunodeficiency Syndrome; a disease of the immune system caused by the virus called HIV.

antibodies: Proteins produced by the body's immune system to fight viruses or other harmful substances.

asymptomatic: Having no symptoms of illness.

blood transfusion: Receiving blood from another person.

condom: A latex covering for the penis that traps semen and prevents it from entering another person's body.

ejaculate: Discharge fluid, especially semen.

hemophilia: A disorder in which a person's blood does not clot, or thicken, properly.

HIV: Human Immunodeficiency Virus; the microscopic organism that causes AIDS.

homosexuality: The emotional and sexual attraction between two people of the same sex.

hospice: A type of care for sick people who are not expected to live more than a few months; includes the services of doctors, nurses, home health aides, social workers, and chaplains.

immune system: The body's set of defenses against disease.

immunodeficient: Lacking a defense against disease.

infectious: Likely to spread from one person to another.

opportunistic infections: AIDS-related illnesses that attack a weakened immune system.

safer sex: Using a condom when having sex.

semen: The male fluid that carries sperm.

symptoms: Signs of illness.

syringe: A device (needle) used to inject drugs into the body.

T cells: White blood cells that fight germs and help protect the body from illness.

virus: A microscopic organism that enters the body and causes diseases.

WHERE TO GO FOR HELP

There are several organizations and hot line numbers you can call to find out more information about AIDS:

United States

National AIDS Hotline
1-800-342-AIDS
1-800-342-2437

National AIDS Hotline in Spanish
1-800-344-SIDA
1-800-344-7432

National AIDS Hotline for the Hearing Impaired
1-800-243-7012

CDC National AIDS Clearing House
P.O. Box 6003
Rockville, MD 20849-6003
1-800-458-5231

Youth Crisis Hotline
1-800-HIT-HOME
1-800-448-4663

National Gay/Lesbian Hotline
1-800-221-7044

National Teen AIDS Hotline
1-800-234-TEEN
1-800-234-8336

Planned Parenthood Federation of America
1-212-541-7800

Canada

The AIDS Committee of Ottawa
207 Queen Street, 4th Floor
Ottawa, ON K1P 6E5
1-613-238-5014

AIDS Hotline
1-613-238-4111

Canadian AIDS Society (Ottawa)
1-613-230-3580

AIDS Committee of Toronto (ACT)
1-416-340-2437

AIDS Coordination Center of Montreal
1-514-873-9890

International

HIV Program
United Nations Development Program
United Nations
New York, NY 10017

FOR MORE INFORMATION

Books

Alexander, Earl, Sheila Rubin, and Pam Sejkora. *My Dad Has HIV.* Fairview Press, 1996.

Anonymous. *It Happened to Nancy: A True Story from the Diary of a Teenager.* Ed. by Beatrice Sparks. Avon Books, 1994.

Crumb, Duane. *Don't Let AIDS Catch You: Straight Talk About AIDS.* American Institute for Teen AIDS Prevention, 1996. (P.O. Box 136116, Fort Worth, TX 70136-6116.)

Dever, Barbara. *AIDS, What Teens Need to Know.* Learning Works, 1996. (P.O. Box 6187, Santa Barbara, CA 93160.)

Draimin, Barbara Hermie, DSW. *Coping When a Parent Has AIDS.* Rosen, 1993.

———. *Working Together Against AIDS.* Rosen, 1994.

Forbes, Anna. *Where Did AIDS Come From?* Rosen, 1996.

Ford, Michael T. *The Voices of AIDS.* Morrow, 1995.

Johnson, Earvin "Magic." *What You Can Do to Avoid AIDS.* Times Books, 1992.

Kelly, Pat. *Coping When You or a Friend Is HIV-Positive.* Rosen, 1995.

Lerman-Golomb, Barbara. *AIDS.* Teen Hot Line Series. Raintree Steck-Vaughn, 1995.

Levert, Maria. *AIDS: A Handbook for the Future.* Millbrook, 1996.

Stewart, Gail B. *People with AIDS.* Lucent, 1996.

White, Ryan, and Anne Marie Cunningham. *Ryan White: My Own Story.* Dial, 1991.

Wiener, L. S., A. Best, P. A. Pizzo, compilers. *Be a Friend: Children Who Live with HIV Speak.* Albert Whitman & Company, 1994.

Government Publications

AIDS: An Expanding Tragedy. The Final Report of the National Commission on AIDS. National Commission on AIDS, 1993. (Available through CDC National AIDS Clearing House.)

Fact Sheets. CDC National AIDS Clearing House, 1996.

Youth & HIV/AIDS: An American Agenda. A Report to the President. Office of the National AIDS Policy, 1996.

Videos

Hope for the Future: Confronting HIV in Children and Adolescents. Produced by AIMS Media, 1993. (9710 DeSoto Ave., Chatsworth, CA 91311-4409.)

"I Have AIDS"—A Teenager's Story. Produced by Children's Television Workshop (V467). CDC National AIDS Clearing House.

Smart Sex. Produced by Lucky Duck Productions (V139); classroom version (V439). CDC National AIDS Clearing House.

INDEX